Master Your Storms,
Master Your Life

T0106496

Master Your Storms, Master Your Life

Mindful Journaling and Sketching for Wisdom and Well-Being

Written and Illustrated by
Teri B. Racey, PA, MA

Part of the *New Mind New Body* series

iUniverse, Inc.
Bloomington

Master Your Storms, Master Your Life
Mindful Journaling and Sketching for Wisdom and Well-Being

Copyright © 2012 by Teri B. Racey, PA, MA

All rights reserved. No part of this book may be used or reproduced by any means, graphic, electronic, or mechanical, including photocopying, recording, taping or by any information storage retrieval system without the written permission of the publisher except in the case of brief quotations embodied in critical articles and reviews.

iUniverse books may be ordered through booksellers or by contacting:

iUniverse
1663 Liberty Drive
Bloomington, IN 47403
www.iuniverse.com
1-800-Authors (1-800-288-4677)

Because of the dynamic nature of the Internet, any web addresses or links contained in this book may have changed since publication and may no longer be valid. The views expressed in this work are solely those of the author and do not necessarily reflect the views of the publisher, and the publisher hereby disclaims any responsibility for them.

The information, ideas, and suggestions in this book are not intended as a substitute for professional advice. Before following any suggestions contained in this book, you should consult your personal physician or mental health professional. Neither the author nor the publisher shall be liable or responsible for any loss or damage allegedly arising as a consequence of your use or application of any information or suggestions in this book.

The book's purpose is to provide you with a means of gaining self-awareness so as to promote deeper levels of self-knowledge which will allow you to make wise and informed choices as a partner in your health care.

Any people depicted in stock imagery provided by Thinkstock are models, and such images are being used for illustrative purposes only.

Certain stock imagery © Thinkstock.

ISBN: 978-1-4759-1156-5 (sc)
ISBN: 978-1-4759-1157-2 (e)

Printed in the United States of America

iUniverse rev. date: 05/11/2012

I express my deep gratitude to all teachers who have shared their wisdom with me—whether that wisdom was shared through experiences of pleasure or pain. I am indebted to them because they have helped me become a stronger and wiser person.

Contents

Acknowledgments

My first and finest teachers were my parents, Chris Battersby and Helen (Buckley) Battersby, and my grandmother Winifred (Mullally) Battersby, all wonderful beacons of love and wisdom. My brothers and sister also shared their wisdom through the everyday joys and challenges experienced in our large and dynamic family. I express my love and gratitude to my sister, Pat, who is my best friend and lifelong counselor; my loving, strong, and steady husband, Joe, who consistently supports my dreams; my amazing daughters, Cara and Andrea, who are loving and wise beacons of light in their own right; my incredible son through marriage, Bryan Fenster; and the entirely wonderful Battersby and Racey clans of which I am so fortunate to be a part.

Special thanks to my personal editorial team: Melissa Cooper Sargent, Cara Fenster, Pat Battersby, and Kevin Witenoff. Special thanks to Chris Elliott for his Illumined Heart drawing that touched the core of our message: walk your path with a wise and loving heart and mind.

Gratitude and Encouragement

I am deeply honored and grateful that you have chosen to invest your valuable time and energy in the use of this journal as a tool for your personal transformation work. May it awaken you to your wise, loving, eternal nature and your fluid connection to universal wisdom.

Master of the Storm

She watched the tornadic winds with awe and fear.
Away from its grip she felt safe and secure.
She did not know that she was of the storm.

Through observation of the storm, she grew in courage, strength,
and in a certainty of the storm's great power and might.
She knew intense fear, yet she knew she was safe and secure.
She did not know that she was of the storm.

Unsatisfied with the distance, she touched the edges of the storm,
experiencing its expelled debris.
She remained fear- and awe-filled, yet again, certain of her safety.
Still, she did not know that she was of the storm.

As her curiosity and strength intensified, she moved closer
and was pulled up into the great vortex, moving up and around,
entangled in the throes of its power.
Yet she knew with a greater certainty than ever before that she was undeniably safe.
Was she of the storm?

She had embraced the storm in full measure and had known great protection.
She now understood that this had always been so.
She was of the storm.

Incorporating its knowledge, she harnessed the storm's power
to draw out darkness, leaving light in its wake.

She is the Master of the Storm.

How You May Benefit from Using This Journal

The "Master of the Storm" poem that provides the framework for this book is the result of the mindfulness journaling and sketching techniques I used to understand my dreams and gain access to my subconscious mind. I found this method of self-discovery so illuminating that I created this book for others who also wish to pursue deep self-exploration by utilizing the principles of mindfulness.

Mindfulness is a discipline that can assist you in becoming more aware of your current ways of interacting with your world and being more present to each moment of your life. It can help you develop the skill of a more relaxed and detached observer so you may identify and better understand ingrained ways of thinking and behaving that keep you reproducing your past. Though we may have limited control over many of the circumstances we find ourselves in, we always have the ability to choose our response. Becoming more conscious of all your reactions and their consequences can help you release ways of reacting that you find create limitations for you so you may respond more effectively in your own behalf. These empowering changes can only take place if you are willing to engage in disciplined, frank self-exploration.

Journaling is a powerful tool for self-discovery. Like the principles of mindfulness, it can also help you uncover and understand emotions, thought patterns, and belief systems that you may not be aware of consciously. This self-discovery process is particularly helpful if you are currently grappling with a health, home, work, or relationship issue.

Becoming aware of your subconscious thoughts, emotions, and behavior patterns by combining the discipline of mindfulness with the journaling and sketching process can provide you with even greater information and insight. Through that richer understanding, you will be better able to advocate in your own behalf and hold greater personal authority over all your affairs. This journal can also provide you with a means to more successfully manage any life challenge as it simultaneously transforms your way of interacting with your world.

It offers a comfortable venue to explore your subconscious mind without limits. In addition, it provides a consistent, structured way to connect you with deep levels of self-knowledge. Knowledge is power.

Self-knowledge empowers you to become an effective self-advocate.

A more complete understanding of how you experience and interact with your world gives you the opportunity to liberate yourself from old ways of thinking and behaving that jail your beautiful spirit. This strong self-leadership allows you to make more empowering choices that help you break "automatic pilot" reactivity cycles that cause you to repeat unhelpful thought and behavior patterns. As you recognize and release these old ways, your greater insight and understanding will guide you to respond more wisely and compassionately to all your life experiences.

The use of this journal will

- support you in developing the discipline of a *scientist of self* so you may observe yourself in the context of a challenge with loving detachment, free of the harsh self-judgment or shame that can limit self-understanding and compassionate self-care;
- help you unravel the complexities of a health or relationship issue so you may calmly and clearly understand it and assert your needs successfully;
- provide a valuable tool in your self-discovery work with a talk therapist and/or group;
- bring automatic and unconscious thoughts, emotions, and behaviors to your conscious awareness so you may release those that no longer serve you and give greater support to those that benefit you now;
- give you the time and emotional space for fruitful self-reflection so you may develop effective self-advocacy strategies;
- help you understand, trust, and work effectively with your intuition;
- provide you with crucial structural distance so you will not be overwhelmed by your emotions and the new awareness that may arise as you continue your exploration; and
- supply a means of uncovering, owning, and expressing your unique and beautiful talents and truth.

Please note that the poem and illustrations found in the journal represent the feminine perspective because they tell the story of my serial storm dreams and how those dreams supported my evolution in consciousness. This poem provides a metaphor for the awakening of the great nurturer within us all, male or female. Walking your path as the master of all your experiences requires the full use of both your feminine and masculine natures. Your masculine nature will shepherd and protect you, while your feminine nature will nurture you and help you manifest your desires.

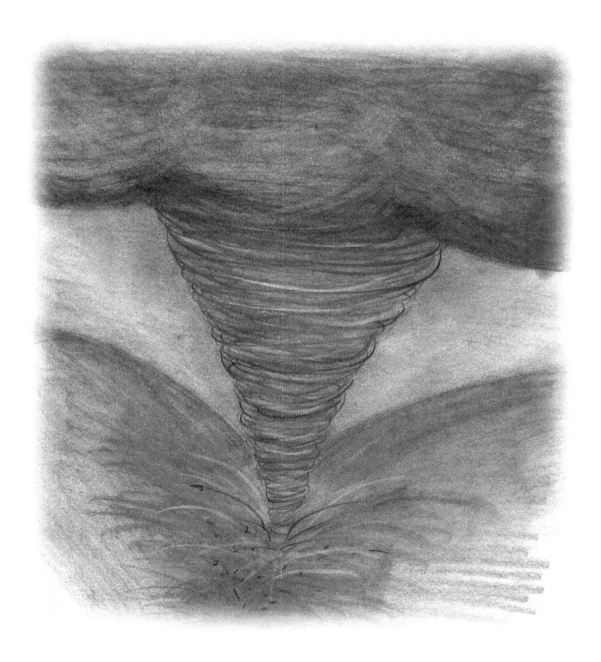

The basic rule of storms is that they continue until the imbalance
that created them is corrected. —*The Day after Tomorrow*

Introduction

The *Master Your Storms, Master Your Life* journal will show you practical ways to overcome challenges by identifying imbalances in thought and action that you come to recognize as factors contributing in some way to your storm. Though you may not have been the author of a particular challenge you face, you most assuredly are the master (or the slave) of your response. Accepting full ownership of your responses to all your interactions with the world leads to self-mastery. Self-mastery is not about conquering the world; it is about having dominion over all your personal affairs so that you are not living based on the opinions or mandates of others. This journal can help you observe and better understand all your reactions as you strive to develop successful strategies for responding that respect your needs and the needs of all others in equal measure. As your self-knowledge grows by reflecting on a challenge and your reactions to it (aided by the mindful writing and sketching process), you will become better able to eliminate ways of interacting that intensify your storms, while simultaneously cultivating ways that bring you a more peaceful, balanced, and joy-filled life.

Walk your path as a Master

The "Master of the Storm" poem, which provides the framework for this journal, was taken from a series of tornado dreams I experienced throughout my life. These dreams and the life situations that spawned them called me to better understand myself and more effectively administer my affairs. The frightening storm dreams compelled my attention to them, and they helped me recognize that whenever I sought to understand and address a challenge, I awakened within myself my own inherent ability to be triumphant. My tornado dreams also helped me to see that my storm can only end when I take the helm to identify and correct those imbalanced thoughts, emotions, and behaviors that gave my storm power. It was through this understanding that I embraced the truth that our challenges are, by design, ours to conquer.

As was true for me, your ability to defeat your storms becomes real to you the moment you acknowledge that you are meant to master them.

When you determine to overcome an obstacle and face a challenge head-on, your inherent personal power ignites and blossoms to offer you support.

Through these experiences, you may even surprise yourself by your ability to assert your needs and desires effectively. This innate self-advocacy provides assistance the moment you embrace the truth that you are the author and shepherd of your every thought, emotion, and behavior. As a child, you were taught by others what was the right and correct way to think, feel, and behave. You were schooled on a book of rules that was specific to your family, cultural, and (perhaps) religious norms. As an adult, if you wish to pursue a course of self-determination, you must revisit these norms to see which of them prevents you from fully expressing your unique truth and valuable talents. This is especially significant to consider for those cognitive, emotional, and behavioral norms that are unpleasant, painful, self-limiting, or a source of shame. It is valuable for you to acknowledge that though these old patterns may still be in play, they are not carved in stone. Though it is crucial to acknowledge your historic thoughts, emotions, and behaviors, it is also important to remind yourself that they need not define how you choose to respond to your current affairs. *You do.*

You are the emoter, not the emotion.
You are the thinker, not the thought.

Each of your thoughts and emotions has value and purpose. They provide important information so you may better understand and more successfully interact with your world.

It is certainly reasonable to avoid or ignore unpleasant or painful thoughts, emotions, and experiences that sidetrack you from enjoying life. Yet every experience of discomfort—no matter how small—provides you with an important "flag" of awareness that helps you notice when your world is imbalanced or there is a potential threat to your health and happiness.

Having a conscious awareness that you are out of balance is invaluable, especially if you desire a life of joyful self-expression.

These disquieting thoughts and emotions are flags of awareness that bring an opportunity to rebalance and reorder your world in a way that will keep you safe and allow you to maintain balanced health and happiness. Flags of awareness can be likened to an *emergency weather alert system* that tells you when a storm is at hand. Responding to an emotional storm effectively takes practice—just as any successful first responder needs practice. Through trial and error, you will learn to respond to these flags of awareness more easily and effectively. Further, through your mindful observations you will discover that the ways you respond seem to calm or deepen your storms.

> You may notice that there are times that you are able to rule your emotions and times that you allow your emotions to rule.

In the latter choice, you will surely deepen your experience of pain; this is not a desirable outcome. It is also essential to make the distinction that ruling your emotions does not mean that you withhold or ignore them. You best rule painful thoughts and emotions by stepping back and mindfully observing them, seeking to examine their expression and understand their meaning. In this choice, you are more likely to gain authority over your emotions, while not ignoring or avoiding them.

Walking with your emotions in this way helps you better understand them, so you may respond in a way that makes it easier to rebalance your current situation and feel more in charge of your life. In this respect, your emergency alert system brings you a powerful gift toward greater self-awareness. The benefits of this gift grow as your greater awareness compels you to search for the source(s) of your unrest, causing you to acquire deeper self-knowledge and discover more effective skills of self-advocacy. Coming to know ourselves more wholly, with all our strengths and vulnerabilities, is crucial if we desire to be the master of our storms.

Self-knowledge is the key to self-mastery

Now you have a rough idea of the benefits you might gain in choosing to use mindful writing and sketching as a tool for cultivating self-knowledge and the skills of self-advocacy. In the next chapter, "What Is Mindful Journaling?" We will explore this unique self discovery process in detail so you may begin the process for yourself.

What Is Mindful Journaling?

Writing in a journal deepens self-understanding and knowledge. When you face a challenge and put your thoughts and emotions down on paper, you are able to step away from them a little and see the bigger picture. You experience even greater clarity when you take the time afterward to review and reflect on what you have written. This conscious, disciplined detachment brings you valuable objectivity. Adding the concept of mindfulness to your journaling and sketching process takes this self-exploration to the next level. It adds the discipline of mindfulness and the creative potential of the right brain to your self-discovery. It brings a consistent structure and sense of calm to your self-investigation. The structure and calm are created by your choice to anchor your mindful observations through your slow, deep breath. Employing this mindfulness process lets you write and sketch with all your senses gathered about you, so you may be fully present to comprehend your entire experience.

While you are mindfully sketching or writing, consciously choose to take slow, deep breaths and intentionally hold your focus on what you are feeling and observing in each moment. This allows you to become fully present to your own unfolding thoughts, emotions, and creative expressions. Engaging this process will also help you remain calm and focused, even to your upsetting thoughts or emotions.

In each moment, allow yourself to observe what is arising within you, consciously breathing in calm and releasing emotional tension with each "out" breath. Let your thoughts and emotions flow freely onto the pages.

During this process, if your focus wanders or seems to avoid or intellectualize a specific thought or emotion, gently shepherd your attention back to your writing and sketching and then express the experience in words or sketches. Disciplining yourself to be engaged and fully present in this way allows your subconscious mind to surface and flow freely. Continue to write or sketch whatever naturally arises in each moment, observing without judgment as you maintain your slow, deep breath work to calm and center you.

It may be helpful to repeat this re-centering exercise as needed during your journaling time:

> As I breathe in slowly—*I welcome in nourishment and calm*
> As I breathe out slowly—*I release stress and tension*

From time to time as you journal, painful thoughts and emotions may arise and feel overwhelming, making it difficult for you to continue your exploration. As this occurs, use your breath work and employ the principles of mindfulness while you journal to help you stay focused and available to observe with loving detachment. This will help you to circumvent the natural inclination to avoid or manage the process. Be mindful and resist the tendency that we all have to intellectualize our thoughts and emotions; this will allow your journaling to be a comprehensive mind/body experience. This disciplined choice allows you to explore your thoughts and emotions unconstrained so you may fully participate in the process without filters. This observer's perspective becomes even more powerful when you fully embrace the mind-set and skills of a "scientist of self" as mindfulness principles suggest. A disciplined scientist observes without judgment or attachment to how things should look or feel.

> As you journal, embrace your scientist of self so you may be present to observe without judging or tweaking emotions or thoughts, thereby letting the writing and sketching process flow unbridled.

Resist the urge to monitor spelling, grammar, or punctuation, which will also limit the free flow of your writing and sketching. This choice takes the intellect out of the gatekeeper role and allows your subconscious mind to more freely share information. This method of automatic or free flow writing and sketching will uncover hidden thoughts and emotions, which may help you dismantle your storm. As you free-flow write, also encourage yourself to freely sketch what you are feeling or sensing. Make a word picture that represents the way you are currently feeling. Begin sketching and just let the sketch reveal and define itself. Notice any judgments you may have, especially toward your artistic abilities, and dismiss them. Avoid the natural inclination to edit your artistic rendering; just let your thoughts and emotions form shapes and colors, and reflect on it only after you feel the sketch is complete.

It is also extremely important to become conscious of how you feel physically as you write and sketch. Choose to stay present and observant in each moment so you may understand how your physical body reacts to your thoughts and emotions.

> Specific emotional and thought patterns are linked with specific physical sensory patterns. Observing both your mind and body experiences during the journaling process is indispensable to greater self-understanding.

For example, you may find that when you explore a certain topic, you feel tightness in your neck and shoulders, experience palpitations, or have queasy feelings in your stomach. Though you may not be consciously aware of it, your physical body is as active a participant in each of your experiences as is your mind. Mind and body are an undeniable team. To work with one is to work with the other; balancing and healing one, is balancing and healing the other.

Transform Your Mind, Transform Your Body

Your body is a powerful teacher. When you quiet the activities of your mind and body—as mindful journaling allows—you can observe the distinct way your body communicates its needs to you, as it also complies with your requests. These physical responses are not separate from your thoughts and emotions; rather they are representative of different aspects of your integrated wholeness. As Dr. Candace Pert documented in her book, *Molecules of Emotion*, your mind is not just in your brain, it's in every cell of your body.

Through solid research such as Dr. Pert presents, we now know that every thought, emotion, and physical experience we have affects our mind/body intimately and entirely. Your mind/body communicates to all aspects of itself through a complex electro/neurochemical network in every moment. Each thought, emotion, or physical experience you have is supported in this way. These complex millisecond mind/body interchanges are recorded and stored in the very cells that are directly involved in the experience. Within these "cellular storage cabinets" are the memories of every communication between your mind and body; this is called cellular memory.

Most cellular memories are not consciously remembered. This is particularly true of painful or fear-filled memories. We often block, bury, or deny these memories in order to avoid experiences of pain. These unpleasant memories can negatively influence how you feel and interact with your world. The continued accumulation of these imbalanced or unpleasant memories can slow or block the dynamic electromagnetic dance needed for each of your body's cells to maintain a state of balance (homeostasis). Your cellular memories accumulate with repetitive thoughts and behaviors; this eventually results in feelings of emotional and physical pain. Held long term, these memories may develop into a chronic mind/body illness that no longer seems to have a logical or discernable cause. This essential mind/body dynamic is vital to keep in mind as you embark on a journey of self-discovery.

> Understanding the concept of cellular memory helps you become more aware of the power you have to create greater mind/body health by engaging in regular emotional housekeeping.

This housekeeping sets you free. To liberate your mind is to liberate your body. Said differently, when you consciously work to shift or transform your thinking, your physical body supports that choice by releasing cellular memories as it simultaneously works to integrate your newly chosen ways of interacting with your world.

This conscious gatekeeping process brings you greater health as it also helps you create a more conscious and effective mind/body partnership. So as you begin your journaling process, regard each thought or feeling that arises within you as an honored guest. Make yourself available to sit with and discover the message that each one brings to you so you may better know yourself and release any self-limiting ways that you identify. In this, your conscious awareness and willingness to introspect become pivotal steps in your journey toward self-mastery. Spend whatever time that seems best for you engaged in the journaling process; usually ten minutes plus per day.

This mindful journaling process can be made even more fruitful if you do the following:

1. Regularly practice "Cultivating Mindfulness" (addendum I). Mindfulness meditation, like mindful journaling, will help you develop the observer's perspective so you may understand your world from the inside out.

2. Use the principles found in the "Four Qualities of Mindfulness" (addendum II) as a guidepost for the journaling process.

3. Practice the "Illumined Heart Deceleration Walking Meditation" (addendum III) to help you feel calm and release overpowering emotions.

4. Listen to *New Mind New Body*, a guided relaxation exercise that will help you release tightness, tension, and cellular memories (Teri B. Racey; available on CD).

How to Begin Mindful Journaling

1. Find a consistent time each day or night so you may journal regularly; consistency of practice will allow the deepest recesses of your subconscious mind to move more easily into conscious awareness.

2. Create a comfortable setting that will allow you to write and sketch freely and express any emotions that may arise.

3. Begin each session by taking several mindful, slow deep breaths to calm and center you. This will help you feel more relaxed as you write and sketch, stimulating deeper insight. If you practice the mindfulness sitting meditation (addendum I) before you begin your writing and sketching session, you will be more relaxed and most open to the flow.

4. Take on your scientist of self and discipline yourself to observe whatever you are feeling, thinking without judgment or attachment so you can write or sketch without restraint.

5. Write or sketch freely, letting your thoughts and emotions fill the pages without monitoring or filtering them. This automatic writing and sketching will help you tap into your subconscious mind and open you to experience thoughts, emotions, and insights of which you are not consciously aware.

6. Discipline yourself to become mindfully aware of any moment that you find yourself monitoring or judging your journaling process and then gently shepherd your attention back to taking slow, deep breaths and journaling.

7. As you become aware of judgments or feelings of anger held toward yourself or others, let them freely flow onto the pages. Review and reflect afterward so you may uncover the seeds of your anger, anxiety, or fear. This will make it easier for you to understand and let go of these toxic emotions. No matter how well justified, these toxic emotions will keep you stuck in a cycle of reactivity that grows stronger with time, creating greater anger, anxiety, and fear within you. Releasing them frees your spirit from this escalating tyranny. Consciously

choose to employ self-compassion and then extend it out to others so you may authentically release these toxic emotions and any unforgiveness you may hold within. Forgiveness frees your spirit!

8. Review and reflect on your words and sketches to gain additional emotional distance and deeper insight. Choose to view your renderings with a compassionate heart and mind. Challenges, by their very definition, are overwhelming, and we respond the best way we are able, considering the emotional and physical resources we have at the time. Most importantly, choosing love and compassion toward yourself and all others frees your spirit to follow more joyful pursuits.

9. As you write and sketch, review and reflect, think about and incorporate the principles of the "Four Qualities of Mindfulness" (addendum II). Strive to apply these principles toward yourself and your situation.

Give More Power to the Process

Remind yourself to remain a disciplined scientist of self even as you review your words and sketches. Loving detachment from complex thoughts and intense emotions will help you see a new view. This perspective can help you to stop reacting to your history and start responding with your new levels of awareness and wisdom. Respect and honor whatever you have written or sketched. See your words and illustrations without the judgments or personal attachments that might bias your review. Remind yourself that you gain wisdom and strength as you address each challenge only if you are able to appreciate its deeper meaning.

> Just as a barnacle-covered oyster shell contains a beautiful pearl within it, so your challenge holds within it the potential for deeper self-knowledge and greater levels of wisdom.

Embrace the pearl and discard the oyster shell. Review your experience as a wisdom seeker. See the unearthed pain as a flag of awareness that points you to an imbalance that you will, in time, successfully correct. Regard yourself with love and compassion. If you find the process too intense, step away from it for a while. Go for a mindfulness walk (addendum III), or engage in some form of physical exercise or another nurturing, joyful diversion. Return to the process when you feel ready to review and reflect again. If you feel you need additional support, call a friend, connect with family, join a support group, and/or make an appointment with a talk therapist or a spiritual advisor in your faith tradition. Look for guidance and support from others, but remind yourself that you must ultimately choose your own course. Choosing to do what others recommend without feeling confident that it is right for you will only create more feelings of disempowerment, which can only prolong and compound your storm.

This journal supports your self-discovery process even further by separating the "Master of the Storm" poem into six empowering steps that will provide a workable structure to help you effectively attend to any personal, professional, health, or relationship challenge.

Six Steps to Success

This journal is intended to support you in the identification of and triumph over your storms through six empowering steps:

1. Become aware.

2. Observe and understand.

3. Own and choose.

4. Look more deeply into the nature of your storm; embrace the full chaos.

5. Demonstrate and celebrate your commitment to change.

6. Walk your path with an illumined heart and mind.

Eagle in a Storm

Did you know that an eagle knows when a storm is approaching long before it breaks?

Sensing the impending storm, the eagle will find a lofty spot and there patiently await the onset of the storm.

When the storm breaks, the eagle spreads its wings and harnesses the storm's energy to lift and soar above it.

While the storm is raging below, the eagle is effortlessly sailing above it, using the very power of the storm as a means of transcending it.

The eagle does not escape the storm.

The eagle does not avoid or deny the storm.

It simply uses the power of the storm to lift itself higher.

Become the eagle of your storm.

You gain strength, courage, and confidence by every experience in which you really stop to look fear in the face.... You must do the thing you think you cannot do. —Eleanor Roosevelt

Master of the Storm

She watched the tornadic winds with awe and fear.
Away from its grip she felt safe and secure.
She did not know that she was of the storm.

Through observation of the storm, she grew in courage, strength,
and in a certainty of the storm's great power and might.
She knew intense fear, yet she knew she was safe and secure.
She did not know that she was of the storm.

Unsatisfied with the distance, she touched the edges of the storm,
experiencing its expelled debris.
She remained fear- and awe-filled, yet again, certain of her safety.
Still, she did not know that she was of the storm.

As her curiosity and strength intensified, she moved closer
and was pulled up into the great vortex, moving up and around,
entangled in the throes of its power.
Yet she knew with a greater certainty than ever before that she was undeniably safe.
Was she of the storm?

She had embraced the storm in full measure and had known great protection.
She now understood that this had always been so.
She was of the storm.

Incorporating its knowledge, she harnessed the storm's power
to draw out darkness, leaving light in its wake.

She is the Master of the Storm.

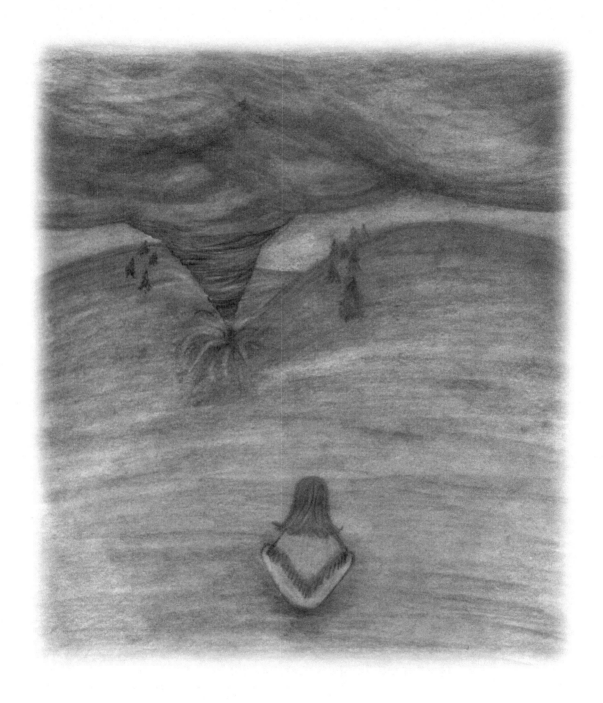

She watched the tornadic winds with awe and fear.
Away from its grip she felt safe and secure. She did not know that she was of the storm.

Step One:
Become Aware

Become a more objective observer of your storm

Life's storms grab your attention by stimulating discomfort, even fear, within you. These feelings tell you there is an imbalance or threat currently present in your world. Though storms speak to a current imbalance that must be corrected, they also serve to wash away the cobwebs, dust, and debris that cloud your perception, making it easier to distinguish the characteristics of the imbalance itself. Gaining insight into the nature of a personal challenge can bring wisdom and feelings of empowerment that lead you to assume greater authority over the challenge and all of your affairs. Mindful journaling helps you view your challenge from an expanded perspective so you may become fully aware of every aspect of your storm and all of your reactions to it. In this greater understanding, you can work with all your reactions and learn how to respond most effectively in your own behalf.

Questions to stimulate your awareness

What is the storm or challenge I am currently facing?

Who are the key players in this storm?

When, where, and how did this storm begin?

Have I experienced similar storms in my past? When? With whom?

What areas of my life are affected by this storm or by my ways of reacting to it?

Enhance the process

Gain deeper self and world awareness. Consciously choose to become aware of your thoughts and reactions to each of your life experiences.

Precede each journaling session by practicing the mindfulness sitting meditation.

The significant problems we have cannot be solved at the same level of thinking we were at when we created them. —Albert Einstein

Journal your thoughts and emotions here

_____

_____

_____

_____

_____

_____

_____

_____

_____

_____

_____

_____

_____

Journal your thoughts and emotions here

_____

_____

_____

_____

_____

_____

_____

_____

_____

_____

_____

Journal your thoughts and emotions here

_____

_____

_____

_____

_____

_____

_____

_____

_____

_____

_____

_____

Journal your thoughts and emotions here

_____

_____

_____

_____

_____

_____

_____

_____

_____

_____

_____

Journal your thoughts and emotions here

_____

_____

_____

_____

_____

_____

_____

_____

_____

_____

_____

_____

Journal your thoughts and emotions here

Draw pictures representing your thoughts and feelings here

Draw pictures representing your thoughts and feelings here

Draw pictures representing your thoughts and feelings here

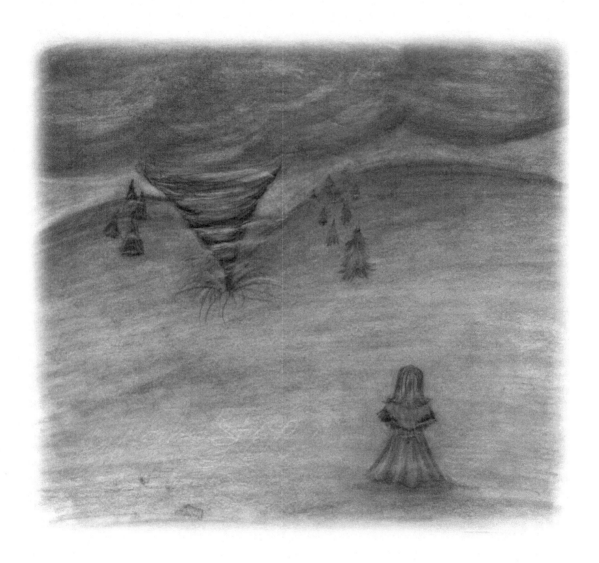

Through observation of the storm, she grew in courage, strength,
and in a certainty of the storm's great power and might.
She knew intense fear, yet she knew she was safe and secure.
She did not know that she was of the storm.

Step Two:
Observe and Understand

You have become more aware of your storm. Hold the focus of your attention on it so you may observe and understand with the mindful detachment that your journaling will provide. To deal effectively with your storm, you must become aware of all aspects of what you are currently facing and understand it on all levels. Mindful journaling will help this process because it provides a method of disciplined self-discovery that allows you to comprehend your circumstances as a scientist. A scientist chooses to observe without judgment or predisposition. This scientific detachment will help you gather information by observing what you see, feel, and sense at some distance, just as if you were watching a television show. Your thoughts and emotions are flags of awareness that alert you to an imbalance and can offer you valuable insight into your situation. Write and sketch what you sense, think, and feel in a free-flowing manner. Review and reflect later on what you have expressed in words and sketches. Trust what your observations and intuition tell you. Honor your emotions but don't allow them to rule; they will help you gain a deeper understanding of yourself and your circumstances, but your ability to reason with compassion should take the leadership position.

Questions to help you observe and understand your storm

What are my thoughts and feelings about this storm? (Allow yourself free-flow expression.)

What old ways of reacting am I bringing to this challenge?

Do these old ways calm or feed the storm? How?

Do I hold resentment or anger toward myself or others? Who? Why?

Am I willing to release these self-limiting thoughts and behaviors?

Enhance the process

Make a list of people and situations that you would like to understand more fully. Take the time to reflect on and explore your relationship to each person or situation that you have listed.

Take on your scientist of self so you may observe and understand your affairs more fully.

Continue practicing the mindfulness sitting meditation to help you stay attentive and focused.

All that we are is a result of what we have thought. —Buddha

Journal your thoughts and emotions here

_____

_____

_____

_____

_____

_____

_____

_____

_____

_____

_____

_____

_____

Journal your thoughts and emotions here

_____

_____

_____

_____

_____

_____

_____

_____

_____

_____

_____

_____

Journal your thoughts and emotions here

_____

_____

_____

_____

_____

_____

_____

_____

_____

_____

_____

Journal your thoughts and emotions here

Journal your thoughts and emotions here

_____

_____

_____

_____

_____

_____

_____

_____

_____

_____

_____

Journal your thoughts and emotions here

_____

_____

_____

_____

_____

_____

_____

_____

_____

_____

_____

Draw pictures representing your thoughts and feelings here

Draw pictures representing your thoughts and feelings here

Draw pictures representing your thoughts and feelings here

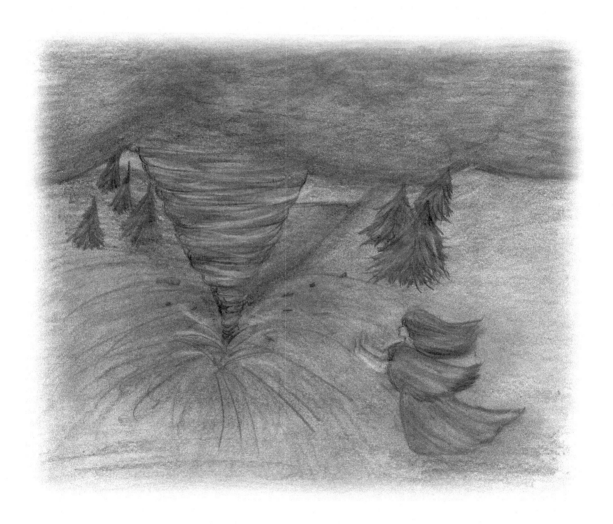

Unsatisfied with the distance, she touched the edges of the storm,
experiencing its expelled debris.
She remained fear- and awe-filled, yet again, certain of her safety.
Still, she did not know that she was of the storm.

Step Three:
Own and Choose

Your observations have brought you to the understanding that this storm is yours to calm. This acceptance of ownership is a pivotal step in mastering your storm and having dominion over all the affairs of your life. Ownership is power. This power gives you the full authority to release emotion, thought, and behavior patterns that no longer serve you. Taking ownership requires a consistent commitment to honesty and integrity, while mindfully shepherding all your reactions so you may become an informed and effective gatekeeper.

Mindful journaling helps you become aware of subconscious self-deceptions and buried experiences that influence your current responses. These old ways or memories are held within the cells of your physical body. It requires a great deal of emotional and physical energy to maintain these ever-compounding memories. Subconsciously holding on to these memories will keep you stuck in patterns of reactivity that jail your beautiful spirit and allow outside influences to make your decisions for you. Journaling will help you identify, own, and choose to release self-limiting ways as you strive to replace them with wiser, more compassionate responses that will bring you greater health, happiness, and the ability to self-determine.

Questions to help you own and choose
Do I feel that I own my ability to self-determine?
Do I expect others to resolve my challenges?
To what extent do I see the wisdom of others as being superior to my own?
Do I contribute in any way to my own experience of voicelessness and powerlessness?

Enhance the process
Make an "ownership list." Identify self-limiting ways of thinking and behaving so you can understand and then modify/release those that you have the ability to influence.

Release unsupportive cellular memories by listening to my guided relaxation meditation CD, *New Mind New Body.*

Continue to engage your scientist of self and practice the mindfulness sitting meditation.

Whatever you resist persists. —Carl Jung

Journal your thoughts and emotions here

_____

_____

_____

_____

_____

_____

_____

_____

_____

_____

_____

_____

Journal your thoughts and emotions here

_____

_____

_____

_____

_____

_____

_____

_____

_____

_____

_____

Journal your thoughts and emotions here

_____

_____

_____

_____

_____

_____

_____

_____

_____

_____

_____

_____

Journal your thoughts and emotions here

_____

_____

_____

_____

_____

_____

_____

_____

_____

_____

_____

_____

_____

Journal your thoughts and emotions here

_____

_____

_____

_____

_____

_____

_____

_____

_____

_____

_____

Journal your thoughts and emotions here

_____

_____

_____

_____

_____

_____

_____

_____

_____

_____

_____

_____

Draw pictures representing your thoughts and feelings here

Draw pictures representing your thoughts and feelings here

Draw pictures representing your thoughts and feelings here

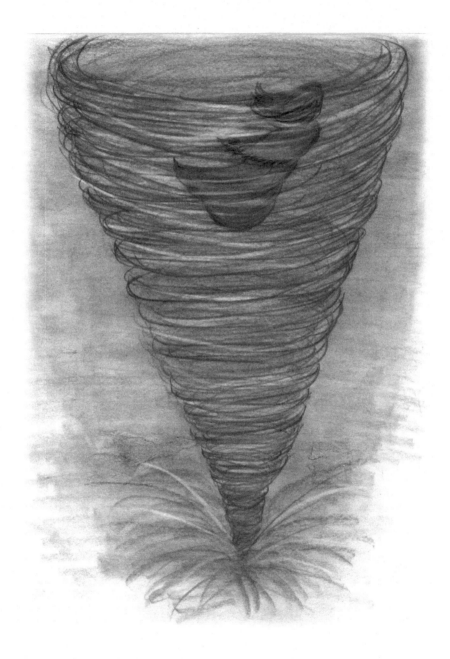

As her curiosity and strength intensified, she moved closer
and was pulled up into the great vortex, moving up and around,
entangled in the throes of its power.
Yet she knew with a greater certainty than ever before that she was undeniably safe.
Was she of the storm?

Step Four:
Look More Deeply into the Nature of Your Storm— Embrace the Full Chaos

Now practiced in mindful awareness and journaling, you have come to understand more deeply about yourself, your storm, and your ability to effectively manage it. You are now able to own your power as a warrior of light—a conscious seeker who pursues wisdom and banishes fear. With greater trust in your own abilities, you can address the core elements of your challenge, especially those foundational ways you deal with adversity in general. Deep self-awareness is the key to lasting empowerment. Reflect on who and/or what brings value and meaning to your life: a belief system, culture, family, friends, or your work. They are your allies in sunshine and shadow. Alternately, you may have discovered that some current key sources of support were actually sapping your power and reinforcing old, imbalanced ways. Let them go or minimize your exposure to them. Place your focus on finding and growing balanced relationships with your true sources of support. Find ways to express your gratitude to them. Seek also to discover *like-minded people* and cultivate new relationships with those that you find respect your unique voice and path.

Questions to help you embrace the full chaos of your storm

What are my sources of support, and how can I connect more fully to them?

What beliefs, relationships, or situations seem to add power to my storm, and how can I modify or release them?

Where can I find like-minded people who support my path and power?

Enhance the process

Make a list of your true support team; find ways to be supportive of them in equal measure.

Make a list of false sources of support and release or modify their impact on you.

Strengthen your support system. Join a support group or begin talk therapy (addendum IV).

Practice the Illumined Heart Deceleration Walking Meditation exercise to help you calm overwhelming thoughts and emotions (addendum III).

Continue to practice the sitting meditation and the *New Mind New Body* guided relaxation CD.

What we hope ever to do with ease, we must learn first to do with diligence.
—Samuel Johnson

Journal your thoughts and emotions here

_____

_____

_____

_____

_____

_____

_____

_____

_____

_____

_____

_____

Journal your thoughts and emotions here

_____

_____

_____

_____

_____

_____

_____

_____

_____

_____

_____

_____

Journal your thoughts and emotions here

_____

_____

_____

_____

_____

_____

_____

_____

_____

_____

_____

_____

Journal your thoughts and emotions here

_____

_____

_____

_____

_____

_____

_____

_____

_____

_____

_____

Journal your thoughts and emotions here

_____

_____

_____

_____

_____

_____

_____

_____

_____

_____

_____

Journal your thoughts and emotions here

_____

_____

_____

_____

_____

_____

_____

_____

_____

_____

_____

Draw pictures representing your thoughts and feelings here

Draw pictures representing your thoughts and feelings here

Draw pictures representing your thoughts and feelings here

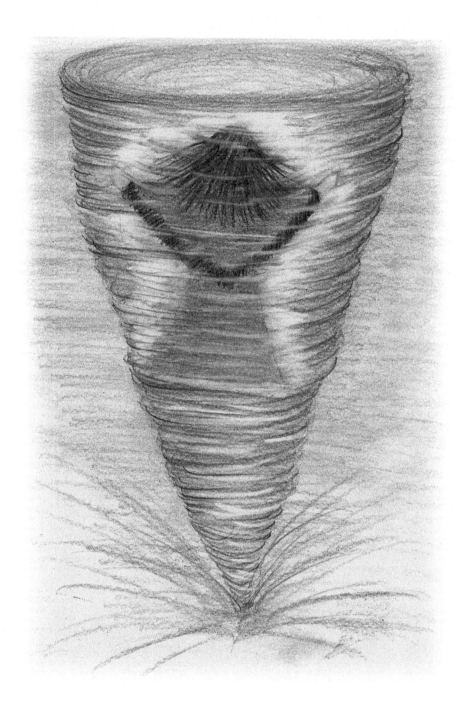

She had embraced the storm in full measure and had known great protection.
She now understood that this had always been so.
She was of the storm.

Step Five:
Demonstrate and Celebrate Your Commitment to Change

You have embraced your storm at its deepest level; dominion over it is now clear. Take time to celebrate your success. Stand strong and resolute in your commitment to change. You have demonstrated your ability to transform your life by consciously altering how you view and interact with your world. Your new mind brings you new life! Compound your success by recognizing that *what you hold as true will be attracted to you*; like attracts like. The understanding of this principle of physics can increase your success only if you carefully and mindfully choose your thoughts and work with all your emotions. Working with this law in this manner can lessen the severity of or even end a future cycle of similar storms.

Take care: this universal law of attraction has a veiled aspect that must also be addressed. Your unconscious painful thoughts and emotions (anger, anxiety, fear, and sorrow) also attract more of the same. For example, memories of anger can create a subtle mind/body addiction cycle, which compels you to seek and entertain relationships and situations that further justify and support your feelings of anger, which create greater unrest and deepen your experience of pain. This makes cultivating self-awareness through mindfulness priceless in helping you identify and release these toxic cellular memories and your attraction to more of the same. As you release these toxic memories, fill the vacated spaces with feelings of compassion and gratitude, and observe the positive shift in how you feel and interact with your world.

Questions to help you demonstrate and celebrate your commitment to change

From what persons or experiences have I learned valuable lessons? How can I apply this wisdom? How can I forgive teachers who shared lessons through pain? How have those lessons changed me? How can I continue to cultivate positive and meaningful personal change?

Enhance the process

Cultivate an "attitude of gratitude" in all your affairs!

Make a list of people who have shared valuable lessons; find an authentic way to thank them.

Forgive those who shared painful lessons and free your spirit from toxic thoughts, emotions, and behaviors.

Continue to practice the sitting and walking meditations and the *New Mind New Body* relaxation CD.

By cultivating one's nature one will return to virtue. —Chuang-Tzu

Journal your thoughts and emotions here

_____

_____

_____

_____

_____

_____

_____

_____

_____

_____

_____

Journal your thoughts and emotions here

_____

_____

_____

_____

_____

_____

_____

_____

_____

_____

_____

_____

_____

Journal your thoughts and emotions here

_____

_____

_____

_____

_____

_____

_____

_____

_____

_____

_____

_____

Journal your thoughts and emotions here

_____

_____

_____

_____

_____

_____

_____

_____

_____

_____

_____

Journal your thoughts and emotions here

_____

_____

_____

_____

_____

_____

_____

_____

_____

_____

_____

_____

Journal your thoughts and emotions here

_____

_____

_____

_____

_____

_____

_____

_____

_____

_____

_____

Draw pictures representing your thoughts and feelings here

Draw pictures representing your thoughts and feelings here

Draw pictures representing your thoughts and feelings here

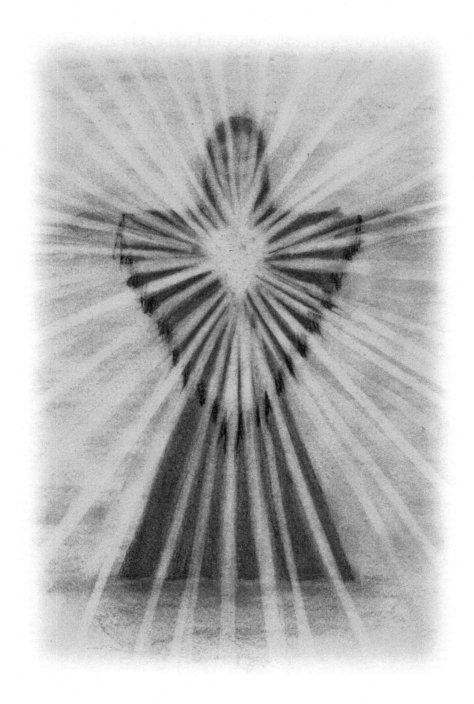

Incorporating its knowledge she harnessed the storm's power to draw out darkness, leaving light in its wake.
She is the Master of the Storm.

Step Six:
Walk Your Path with an Illumined Heart and Mind

You have demonstrated your ability to end your storm and move toward self-mastery; let the process continue and expand within you. Consciously walk your path with a wise, loving heart and mind as you apply your newfound knowledge and abilities. Because you now embrace the wisdom found within your storm, its purpose has been fulfilled. Just as you would naturally discard the oyster shell once you hold the pearl, release your emotional experience of the storm once you hold the knowledge. The storm's end also brings an opportunity for you to share your acquired wisdom through compassion. Wisdom and love compound within you by their expression. Be mindful as you offer support to others; respect that they must walk their paths in their own unique ways. Convey affection and insight through the example of your life or under circumstances where you are specially invited to share. This option sends the essential message that you acknowledge others' abilities to effectively address their challenges and be the masters of their own lives. Bring your blossoming wisdom and compassion to every area of your life; in each mindful moment, find meaningful ways to grow and express your illumined heart and mind.

Questions to help you nurture your illumined heart and mind

How can I use my tools of mindfulness to bring compassion and insight to new challenges?

How can I give meaningful support to others as they move through their storm(s)?

Enhance the process

Continue to use the tools of mindfulness daily.

Continue to practice the sitting and walking meditations and the *New Mind New Body* relaxation CD.

Revisit these pages to work through each new challenge.

Give back to those who supported you and to those facing a struggle you have now mastered.

Strive to approach each moment mindfully, with a wise and compassionate heart and mind.

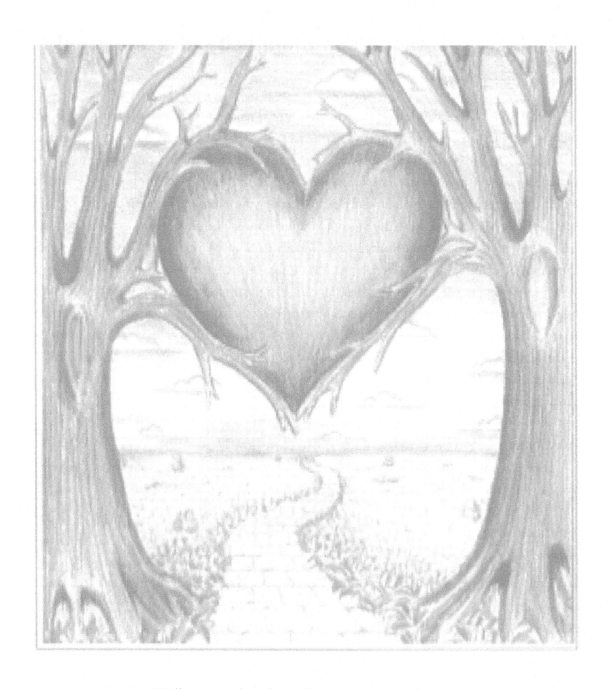

Walk your path with an illumined heart and mind.

The man of perfect virtue, wishing to be established himself, seeks also to establish others; wishing to be enlarged himself, he seeks also to enlarge others. —Confucius

Journal your thoughts and emotions here

_____

_____

_____

_____

_____

_____

_____

_____

_____

_____

_____

Journal your thoughts and emotions here

_____

_____

_____

_____

_____

_____

_____

_____

_____

_____

_____

Journal your thoughts and emotions here

_____

_____

_____

_____

_____

_____

_____

_____

_____

_____

_____

Journal your thoughts and emotions here

_____

_____

_____

_____

_____

_____

_____

_____

_____

_____

_____

_____

_____

Journal your thoughts and emotions here

_____

_____

_____

_____

_____

_____

_____

_____

_____

_____

_____

Journal your thoughts and emotions here

_____

_____

_____

_____

_____

_____

_____

_____

_____

_____

_____

_____

Draw pictures representing your thoughts and feelings here

Draw pictures representing your thoughts and feelings here

Draw pictures representing your thoughts and feelings here

Addendum I
Cultivating Mindfulness

Author's Note:

Many wise teachers have devoted their lives to practicing and teaching mindfulness. Thich Nhat Hanh, Jon Kabat-Zinn, and Saki Santorelli are among my teachers. I honor and express my gratitude to them and all other beacons of light for the vast healing influence their work has on human consciousness.

I have, over the past several decades, taught the concepts of mindfulness meditation to countless individuals and groups with compelling results. I have witnessed great personal transformations for those who practice regularly. These individuals have been able to significantly reduce or eliminate symptoms of chronic pain, insomnia, anxiety, and depression. Those individuals who meditate regularly also found that they cope more effectively with chronic medical conditions. I have also observed many who have made empowering changes in their relationships with others. These results were so consistent and dramatic that I changed the entire focus of my professional practice. If you choose to devote time to practice the mindfulness sitting meditation, you will also experience welcome and empowering changes in your mind and body as well as in your ways of interacting with your world.

Health, a light body, freedom from cravings, a glowing skin, sonorous voice, fragrance of body: these signs indicate progress in the practice of meditation.
—Shvetashvatara Upanishad

What Is Mindfulness?

Mindfulness is the ancient Buddhist discipline of consciously choosing to be fully present and aware of all that is in your world in each moment, whether that moment is pleasant or unpleasant. The discipline of mindfulness calls you to consciously engage your mind and all your senses in the observation of each moment with an unwavering commitment to honesty and integrity. The practice of mindfulness meditation is the means through which you cultivate this moment-to-moment awareness; it is how you strengthen your "mindfulness muscles."

The discipline of mindfulness also allows you to expand your awareness into your higher consciousness, which is your connection to the infinite wisdom of the universe. Here, in this present moment, is the only aspect of the time/space continuum where you are able to consciously touch this cosmic flow. Mindfulness also invites you to observe each moment with a beginner's mind; to become still and view your inner and outer worlds with the patience, trust, and the curiosity of a child who has not yet learned how to judge, qualify, and quantify her world.

> Mindfulness meditation is a technique that allows you to investigate life from the inside out rather than the outside in.

Mindful awareness of your thoughts, emotions, and interactions with your world are the keys to conscious living. Self-knowledge and mastery come from a mindful decision to listen to your inner dialogue and observe your thoughts, emotions, and interactions with your world without the judgment that might cloud or bias fruitful self-reflection. This observational process should include a choice not to include predispositions or attachments in your discovery process. Like judgment, attachment to any outcome can limit your ability to experience an expanded worldview. Employing the discipline of mindfulness will also allow you to hold a position of strong self-leadership so you may tap into and harness the information and resources that will help you engage in wise and compassionate decision making.

Establishing Your Time and Location of Practice

Practice the mindfulness sitting meditation for a thirty-minute period of time, twice a day. If you cannot allocate this much time, it is more helpful to practice some than none. Shorter practice periods can still be fruitful. Even five minutes of slow, deep breathing with your eyes closed can bring greater nourishment to your mind and body.

Next find a comfortable and quiet place where you will not be interrupted. The mindfulness sitting meditation is best practiced in the seated position to help you stay alert; you might more easily fall asleep if you practice while lying down. If you are unable to sit comfortably due to health-related issues, it will not create significant limitations by adjusting your position to comfort. You may find it helpful to begin your session in an area specifically designated for meditation.

You may prefer to practice while sitting in bed, perhaps just before your night's sleep and then again upon awakening. Set your alarm to awaken you thirty minutes early. When you awaken, simply sit up, reset your alarm for your designated wake-up time, and begin your meditation. While this plan will leave you with sixty minutes less sleep each night, you will sleep more deeply and awaken more refreshed. If you find that you fall asleep while practicing in your comfy bed, the meditation is not likely to help bring greater clarity to your everyday affairs. The practice of mindfulness meditation is a discipline wherein you focus and center your mind while you endeavor to maintain a relaxed and alert consciousness.

This discipline allows you to observe your thoughts in a detached manner so you may experience clarity, insight, and deepen self-knowledge. In order for this dynamic process to occur and strengthen within you, you must be an active and conscious participant in the process. This self-observation aspect of practice will allow you to become a compassionate and detached observer of all of your thoughts, emotions, and ways of interacting with your world. You will become a disciplined scientist of self. As you cultivate this level of self-awareness by embracing the observer's perspective, you will be available to choose new ways of interacting with your world that naturally bring you greater health and happiness. These new ways of responding will eventually become the manner in which you address all of your affairs. You will become able to mindfully respond to each new situation as it arises rather than react mindlessly from your history. This fresh, more empowered way of interacting with your world requires discipline, which practicing the mindfulness sitting meditation will help you cultivate. Before your first mindfulness sitting meditation, allow me to outline the basic mechanics of a meditation session.

Highlights of the Mindfulness Sitting Meditation

1. Assume a seated position in a quiet, comfortable place where you will not be disturbed.

2. Close your eyes; relax and gather all of your senses.

3. Focus your attention on the ebb and flow of your breath with all your senses engaged so you will be entirely available to observe this dynamic process in each moment.

4. Slow and deepen your breath as you continue to focus your attention on its flow by observing the movements of your lungs, chest, and abdomen.

5. As you observe the flow of your breath, also observe the flow of your thoughts. Resist the natural tendency to judge or engage them.

6. Discipline yourself to maintain the focus of your attention and your observations, noting but not engaging the activities of your mind.

7. Whenever you find yourself drawn to a particular thought, emotion, physical sensation, or outside distraction, choose to gently—and without judgment—return your focus to the observation of your breath.

Mindfulness Sitting Meditation: Instructions

I suggest that before you begin your first mindfulness sitting meditation session, you read through these instructions. This will familiarize you with the process and make it easier for you to relax into your meditation.

The mindfulness sitting meditation exercise begins with a decision to close your eyes with the intention to relax your mind and body and take on the observer's perspective, engaging your scientist of self.

This decision ignites an imperceptible cascade of physiologic changes within your mind and body that support your decision to relax. Observe as a scientist—without judgment or attachment—how your body responds; especially how your chest and abdomen expand and contract as you breathe *in* and *out* through your nose. With your eyes remaining closed, feel how your lungs expand as you welcome in each breath and how they contract each time you release each breath. Always begin your session by observing your lung capacity to help you develop greater awareness of your physical body.

If you are like most people, your lung capacity is frequently restricted to the top half, one-third, or even one-quarter of your lungs. This is the short, shallow breath of stress, which is—in our fast-paced and demanding world—the norm for most of us. Many times, without being consciously aware of it, you may even forget to breathe at all! Once you acknowledge the range and flow of your breath as it is right now, allow yourself to gently welcome a deeper, more nourishing breath into your lungs. Keep in mind that it is best not to push or force your lungs to open beyond comfort, as this creates its own stress on your body. Just allow yourself to welcome a slower, deeper breath in to a comfortable capacity.

Imagine, if you so desire, that your source of infinite love and nourishment—the breath of life—is flowing to and through you with each breath you take. Become attentive to this elegant system of nourishment and cleansing within as you welcome fresh air into your lungs and release stale air. Notice how your mind's intention to breathe more slowly and deeply is supported by your body's innate sympathetic response. This is evidence of the sacred teamwork between your mind and body.

> Imagine nourishing every cell in your body more completely with each *in* breath, and releasing accumulated tension and stress with each *out* breath.

Observe your slow, deep breaths and notice your body's ability to work in harmony and compliance with your intention. This brings you an awareness of the well-designed intelligence of your body, and the nourishing and cleansing qualities of your breath. Because you have consciously chosen to relax, and have intentionally slowed and deepened your breath, your body's physiologic relaxation response releases an electro/neurochemical flow that supports you in achieving your desire for relaxation. Your slow, deep breaths stimulate your parasympathetic nervous system to relax you. Your body conforms further to your intentional request by slowing your brain waves and releasing designated neurochemicals that promote relaxation in every cell of your body.

> As you continue to breathe slowly and deeply, become aware of the ebb and flow of your breath, letting your breath take on its own natural rhythm.

Once your breath assumes a more relaxed ebb and flow, refocus your awareness on the movement and range of your breath only when you notice that your attention has wandered. It is typical during a practice session to become more aware of distracting thoughts, emotions, outside noises, or physical sensations. This is the norm for most of us because we frequently experience a fragmented multitasking mind based on the multiplicity of our daily demands.

> The discipline of mindfulness can help you move away from an unsettled, chaotic mind and develop greater calm and focus.

Your meditation practice helps you accomplish this worthy goal as follows: each time your mind wanders and focuses on a distraction and you choose to gently return your focus to your breath, you form and strengthen new neurological pathways in your brain that will, with repeated practice, bring you a greater ability to focus in all your affairs.

Interestingly, it is the very loss of your focus that provides the means through which you will eventually achieve greater focus! Be mindful that your loss of focus through the engagement of these distractions may also quicken your breath and increase your stress hormones. A conscious return to a slower, deeper breath is necessary to reverse this trend. These distracting thoughts and emotions are called *mind chatter*; mindfulness practitioners call this state of mind the *monkey mind*.

> The more stress neurochemicals you have flowing in your body from a hectic and demanding experience or day, the more mind chatter you will experience during a given practice session.

When the level of mind chatter is high during your practice, the session will naturally be more challenging. Be gentle and patient with yourself. Each time you observe that your awareness is fixed on a distraction, resist the tendency to judge or become frustrated with yourself; simply shepherd your attention back to the observation of your breath.

> Refocusing your attention on your slow, deep breathing process instead of your mind chatter will help you become more calm and centered as it simultaneously lessens the flow of stress neurochemicals and stimulates the production of your relaxation neurochemicals.

It may be helpful to imagine these distractions as if they are fish swimming by you in a gently flowing river. Each fish represents a thought or emotion you become consciously aware of, while the river represents the ongoing flow of your consciousness. Endeavor to observe the many fish and the continuing flow of the river as you discipline yourself to avoid the natural inclination to focus on a particular fish (thought or emotion).

This choice helps you more fully understand all the fish (all your thoughts and emotions), the dynamic flowing river (your dynamic mind), and your experience of them. Alternately, you might choose to view these distractions as words displayed on a passing road sign that might attract your attention as you drive by them. To keep safe, it is important that your focus remains on the road and not on the road signs. The road signs can be likened to the potentially distracting thoughts that might draw your attention to them and the expanding road compared to the flow of your breath. Choosing to see the road signs with your peripheral vision can be compared to observing your mind chatter without engaging it; keeping your focus on the road can be compared to keeping your focus on your breath work.

> Keeping your focus on your breath is as helpful to growing your meditation practice as keeping your focus on the road is helpful to keeping you safe while you drive.

Consider additionally, that whenever you experience a lot of mind chatter, it is understandable to become frustrated and want to force the chatter out of your mind. Though reasonable, this choice is not helpful to the cultivation of a calm and centered mind because this very process can ignite your stress neurochemicals and further accelerate your feelings of frustration and anxiety. This cause and effect can be explained by a law of physics: "For every action, there is an equal and opposite reaction." In other words, if you push a thought out of your mind it will inevitably push back and become more compelling. You have inadvertently chosen to engage the thought or emotion in a tug-of-war! Choose instead to disengage this process by becoming aware of it and letting it go so you can return the focus of your attention on the observation of your breath. Nevertheless, each distraction has value; it provides self-awareness of what is moving through your conscious mind presently and can also serve as a reminder to hold the focus of your attention on your breath so you do not "feed" the distraction.

In this way, the distraction itself serves to strengthen your "mindfulness muscles" and fortify your overall discipline. As your practice session continues, remind yourself to take on the all-important disciplines of nonjudgment and nonattachment (your scientist of self) toward what you are feeling or experiencing.

> Meditation is a dynamic process. In each moment, you observe the activities of your mind and body while maintaining your focus on your breath; then you find that you are drawn away to and have engaged a distraction; then your awareness of this calls you to gently return your focus to the flow of your breath.

This ongoing, dynamic cognitive dance is the fundamental concerto in play in a mindfulness meditation. It is a process that is indispensable if you wish to utilize mindfulness as a vehicle toward self-discovery and mastery. Once your practice session is complete, it is also valuable and supportive to the cultivation of mindfulness to resist the natural tendency to critique or judge your sitting meditation as good or bad, right or wrong. Let your experience simply inform you of where your thoughts and emotions are at this moment so you may know more deeply about your own multifaceted, vibrant nature. Further, because it is desirable to have a peaceful and quiet mind at the end of a meditation session, you may believe that this is a necessary endpoint in order to call the session a success. This is not the case.

> Your session is wholly beneficial to you if you were simply able to refocus your attention on a slow, deep breath whenever you were distracted.

Remind yourself that this methodology helps you develop the observer's mind so you may receive and process information in a more focused, calm, and expanded manner. Remember, each time you return your attention from a distraction back to the observation of your breath, you are creating new neuro-circuitry and reinforcing new ways your brain will identify and process incoming cognitive/sensory data. With repeated practice, this novel process will become an ingrained habit, allowing you to view your life experiences from a calmer, more centered, and expanded perspective. Employ this mindfulness sitting meditation practice for the suggested thirty minutes, twice each day.

Post-Meditation Reflection

Take a moment to reflect after your sitting session. At this point, you may wish to begin your writing and sketching and use that process as a means of reflecting. Know that your meditation practice will bring you a new mind—an expanded and more balanced way of viewing and interacting with your world. This new approach can support you in responding to your challenges through calm reflection. Remind yourself to review your session without judgment, and that the amount of mind chatter you experienced in your session is proportionate to the number of stress neurochemicals flowing through your body just prior to your session.

A chaotic day or experience will always result in an unsettled mind.

Greater levels of stress neurochemicals naturally flow through your body whenever you have a trying experience or day. If you find your mind chatter is consistently overwhelming in your meditation sessions, it may be beneficial to change the time or venue of practice, practice an Illumined Heart Deceleration Walking Meditation (addendum III), or consider some yogic stretches (or a full class) before you sit. Movement meditations like the walking meditation or yoga are often used as a precursor to the sitting meditation.

In fact, the original intent of yoga was to prepare the body, mind, and spirit for the sitting meditation practice. Because yoga, walking meditations, and other movement meditations allow us to engage more body systems in the focusing process, they result in a stronger neurochemical shift, making it easier to calm the activity of the mind.

Alternately, consider practicing your meditation upon awakening, when the mind is usually quieter; this may allow you to experience a deeper level of relaxation within your practice session. Feeling the benefits of your meditation practice is an important reinforcement, which promotes regular practice. Practice is always challenging at first, but immeasurably rewarding. As your experience increases, it will become easier for your mind to remain peaceful for longer periods of time. As this occurs, you will also begin to feel a deeper sense of relaxation outside of your practice sessions, which will help you deal more easily and effectively with your everyday challenges.

Mindfulness in Your Everyday World

Bringing the discipline of mindfulness into your daily affairs can also support great transformations in your relationships. It helps you engage in honest, fruitful, emotional, and behavioral housekeeping, creating a more welcome and comforting quality to your interactions with others. When you are able to nurture a loving and kind attitude toward yourself, it becomes easier to extend love and kindness to others. We are often in very stressful situations, making it more challenging to maintain equanimity within ourselves and in our relationships. External stressors must produce stress neurochemicals within your mind and body because it is how your body is designed to support you in successfully coping with perceived threats.

This valuable neurochemical support system also assists you in accomplishing your daily demands. Equally important to note is that this demand-driven physiologic influx of supportive stress hormones often maintains a hyperalert status that can be very challenging to quiet and reverse. Be patient and understanding with yourself; your attempts at achieving balance and equanimity may be initially difficult, especially if you are accustomed to participating in and seeing rapid responses.

Acknowledge that your impeccably well-designed body provides you with an excitation and relaxation neurochemical feedback system intended to support your needs, as it also strives to seek and maintain equilibrium or homeostasis. Though the excitation support system is an automatic process, your body's ability to achieve relaxation requires your conscious support.

> Your internal stress responder is always at the ready, but you must initiate occasions for rest, relaxation, and recovery.

If you are like most people, you are frequently unable to take your three "Rs" as often as is best for balanced health. Because of this, sleep time may be the only opportunity your body and mind have to rest, relax, and restore. This is often not enough, especially if you regularly experience some form of insomnia. You must consciously and consistently create circumstances to address this vital need your mind and body have for rest, relaxation, and restoration. Your mind/body by its very design seeks balance. If you do not find effective ways to address this call for homeostasis, sheer exhaustion or system breakdown—in the form of an illness or injury—will force the issue. In other words, if you do not create occasions to rest, relax, and recover, you will be faced with a situation where your body and mind will no longer be able to function effectively.

Meditation practice provides an important and beneficial way for us to tap into our relaxation neurochemicals and consciously promote rest, relaxation, and recovery.

Becoming consciously aware of your current level of stress reactivity, as is evidenced by your level of fatigue or other mind/body symptoms of overload, helps to remind you to restore yourself through relaxation activities such as mindfulness meditation.

Through mindful attention, you can identify and correct your mind/body imbalances before they create significant, lasting physical and emotional storms.

You now have a valuable tool to observe your world more entirely, like a scientist of self, from a place of safety that is your operations center within; therein you can correct imbalances that keep you from greater health and happiness.

Addendum II
Four Qualities of Mindfulness

The Quality of Compassionate Listening

Listening completely through a mind and heart filled with love to both our inner dialogue and the words others share with us can heal deep wounds. When we listen compassionately, we connect on a deep soul level and bring tribute to the communion of souls that is free of judgments or a need to problem solve. This level of listening brings validation to the experiences of the speaker and acknowledgment to the inherent ability we all have to access infinite wisdom to resolve our conflicts and challenges. Compassionate listening also brings benefits to the listener. The realization that listening with compassion provides the highest level of support and action releases the listener from the obligation to "do something." This active listening encourages the essential self-advocacy needed to effectively engage in our soul work. Through mindfulness we can learn to listen more entirely to ourselves and others and experience deep understanding.

The Quality of Deep Understanding

As we become more adept at compassionate listening, deep understanding of ourselves and others will develop. Perceiving a person or situation beyond the understandable barriers of fear and judgment and the troublesome interactions that issue from them is easier when we seek deep understanding. In a desire to cultivate the quality of deep understanding, we open ourselves to the recognition and acceptance that these emotions and reactions to our world are part of our human experience. Compassionate listening brings deeper levels of understanding as deeper levels of understanding engender greater compassion and generate a desire for action.

The Quality of Compassionate Action

As we open ourselves to experience greater understanding through compassionate listening, we are naturally drawn into compassionate action. We desire at this point to involve ourselves in work that will lessen our suffering and the suffering of others. Compassionate listening and deep understanding help us formulate a viable plan of action that will prove useful in lessening or ending individual and collective experiences that produce suffering.

The Quality of Being Present

The quality of being fully present in each moment to ourselves and others is the best gift we can offer. Mindfulness practice helps us stay the course and remain fully present for the pleasures and pains of our shared human existence. This allows us to become more able to be fully present for the joy and suffering that exist simultaneously within ourselves and our world. As we become fully present to incidents of suffering, we can consciously work to lessen or eradicate them, allowing joy to flow more freely. Disciplining ourselves to be mindfully present in each moment is how we become able to listen with compassion, gain deep understanding, and act in an informed, wise, and compassionate manner on behalf of all life.

Addendum III
Illumined Heart Deceleration Walking Meditation

Phase One

Pick a pleasant and peaceful location for your walk. Observe and identify the rate of your current thoughts or mind chatter. Attempt to match the speed of your thoughts with the speed of your walk. For example, if you are experiencing a lot of mind chatter, start out by walking as fast as you gauge that you are thinking. (Please first consult your health-care practitioner if you have any physical health conditions.) Be mindful of any physical discomfort or limitation you may have and adjust your pace accordingly. As you start your walk, at whatever pace you have chosen, observe the movements of your mind, body, and breath.

> Observe: How does your body feel? How are your legs and arms moving? Is there any difference in strength and flexibility between the right and left sides of your body? What is the range and flow of your breath?

Allow yourself to make adjustments in your breathing and body movements so you can match them to the speed or level of your mind chatter. In other words, try to merge your mind, body, and breath to the same speed as your thoughts and emotions. It might be helpful to give a rough number to the level of your mind chatter by comparing it to the rotations per minute of an old record-player turntable.

> Ask yourself, What is my current "turntable thought speed" or the rotations per minute (RPMs) of my mind chatter? Use the slow, $33\frac{1}{3}$; medium, 45; or fast, 78 rotations per minute as a rough gauge.

For example, if you assess that your mind chatter is at 78 RPMs, adjust your walking pace so it matches that speed. Then harness your breath work to join the mind/body process at the same speed. As you continue to walk, keep your attention and focus on the expansion and contraction of your lungs, and all the movements of your body. Observe your breath, body movements, and thoughts mindfully as a scientist of self. Continue at this pace until you sense that your mind chatter, body movements, and breath are working in harmony (all at the same speed).

Phase Two

Now that you have matched the current pace of your mind and body with your breath work, you can begin the deceleration portion of this exercise and slow your pace down a bit (five to ten RPMs at a time). Slowing your pace will instigate the process of dialing down your stress neurochemicals, which will force a more rapid neurochemical shift than is possible through a mindfulness sitting meditation alone. (Alternately, if you are feeling exhausted, picking up your pace and the cadence of your breath will allow your excitation neurochemicals to give you a boost.) Continue to mindfully adjust your pace, downshifting your "gears" every five or so minutes until you are at 33⅓ RPMs and feel more relaxed and alert.

Phase Three

Now more relaxed, allow the focus of your attention to shift to the world around you. Use all of your senses. Become mindfully aware of your environment. Listen to the sounds of nature or the ambiance of your walking setting. Take in the shapes, colors, and fragrances around you with all your senses—even the air and sun as they touch your skin. What are your thoughts and feelings as you tune in to nature? Be fully present to yourself in this place, at this moment, and engage it as if you are seeing it for the first time. The awareness that these experiences bring to you may stimulate many thoughts and emotions. When you find yourself focusing on experiences of the past or concerns of the future, gently regather your senses through a slow, deep breath and recommit yourself to fully engage yourself in this moment.

Enjoy this exercise for at least ten to fifteen minutes or as long as you desire.

This deceleration exercise can also be accomplished using a treadmill or stationary bike when circumstances do not allow an outdoor walk. Whenever possible, make every effort to walk outdoors so you may experience the healing and rejuvenating effects that only nature can bring.

Addendum IV
Reading and Resource List

Books

Beattie, Melody. 1987. *Codependent No More*. Minnesota: Hazelden.

Benson, Herbert, MD. 1985. *Beyond the Relaxation Response*. New York: HarperCollins.

————. 1976. *The Relaxation Response*. New York: Berkley Books.

————. 1997. *Timeless Healing: The Power and Biology of Belief*. New York: Fireside Books.

Branden, Nathaniel, PhD. 1992. *The Power of Self-Esteem*. Florida: Health Communications, Inc.

Chopra, Deepak, MD. 1993. *Ageless Body, Timeless Mind*. New York: Harmony Books.

————. 1989. *Quantum Healing*. Bantam Books.

Dossey, Larry, MD. 1996. *Prayer Is Good Medicine*. New York: HarperCollins.

Easwaran, Eknath. 1990. *Words to Live By*. Nilgiri Press.

Ferrini, Paul. 1994. *Love Without Conditions*. Massachusetts: Heartways Press.

————. 1996. *The Silence of the Heart*. Massachusetts: Heartways Press.

————. 1991. *The Twelve Steps of Forgiveness*. Massachusetts: Heartways Press.

Foundation for Inner Peace. 1976. *A Course in Miracles*. California: Foundation for Inner Peace.

Gerber, Richard, MD. 2000. *A Practical Guide to Vibrational Medicine*. New Mexico: HarperCollins.

Gibran, Kahlil. 1923. *The Prophet*. New York: Alfred Knopf, Inc.

Goldsmith, Joel S. 1956. *The Art of Meditation*. New York: HarperCollins Publishers.

Hanh, Thich Nhat. 2001. *Anger: Wisdom for Cooling the Flames*. New York: Riverhead Books.

————. 1998. *Interbeing: Fourteen Steps for Engaged Buddhism*. California: Parallax Press.

————. 1975. *The Miracle of Mindfulness*. Massachusetts: Beacon Press.

————. 1991. *Peace Is Every Step*. United States of America: Bantam Books.

Kabat-Zinn, Jon, PhD. 1990. *Full Catastrophe Living*. New York: Random House.

————. 1994. *Whenever You Go There You Are*. New York: Hyperion.

————. 2011. *Mindfulness for Beginners: Reclaiming the Present Moment and Your Life*. Colorado: Sounds True.

Lama, Dalai. 2001. *An Open Heart: Practicing Compassion in Everyday Life*. United States of America: Little, Brown & Company.

Lama, Dalai and Howard Cutler, MD. 1998. *The Art of Happiness*. New York: Penguin.

Lerner, Harriet, PhD. 1985. *The Dance of Anger*. New York: HarperPerennial.

Locke, Steven, MD. 1987. *The Healer Within*. Oklahoma: Signet.

Merton, Thomas. 1951. *Ascent to Truth*. New York: Harcourt, Inc.

Moore, Thomas. 1996. *The Education of the Heart*. New York: HarperCollins.

Millman, Dan. 1984. *The Way of the Peaceful Warrior*. California: H. J. Kramer, Inc.

Myss, Caroline, PhD. 1996. *Anatomy of a Spirit*. New York: Three Rivers Press.

_____. 2004. *Invisible Acts of Power*. New York: Free Press.

_____. 1997. *Why People Don't Heal and How They Can*. New York: Harmony Books.

Naparstek, Belleruth. 1994. *Staying Well with Guided Imagery*. New York: Warner Books.

Orloff, Judith, MD. 2000. *Intuitive Healing*. New York: Random House.

Oz, Mehmet, MD. 1998. *Healing from the Heart*. New York: Penguin.

Pert, Candice, PhD. 1997. *Molecules of Emotion: Why You Feel the Way You Feel*. New York: Scribner.

Renard, Gary. 2002. *The Disappearance of the Universe*. California: Hay House.

Rossman, Martin L., MD. 1987. *Healing Yourself*. California: H.J. Kramer.

Ruiz, Don Miguel. 1997. *The Four Agreements*. California: Amber-Allen Press.

_____. 1999. *The Mastery of Love*. California: Amber-Allen Press.

Santorelli, Saki, PhD. 1999. *Heal Thy Self*. New York: Random House.

Sternberg, Esther, MD. 2001. *The Balance Within*. New York: W. H. Freeman and Co.

Weil, Andrew, MD. 2001. *Eating Well For Optimal Health*. New York: HarperCollins.

_____. 1995. *Spontaneous Healing*. New York: Alfred A. Knopf, Inc.

Williams, Mark, PhD, John Teasdale, PhD, Zindal Segal, PhD, Jon Kabat-Zinn, PhD. 2007. *The Mindful Way through Depression: Freeing Yourself from Chronic Unhappiness*. New York: Guilford Press.

Williamson, Marianne. 1992. *A Return to Love*. New York: HarperPerennial.

CDs

Kabat-Zinn, Jon, PhD. 2005. *Guided Mindfulness Meditation*. Sounds True.

_____. 2006. *Mindfulness for Beginners* (audio book). Sounds True.

_____. 2009 *Mindfulness Meditation for Pain Relief: Guided Practices for Reclaiming Your Body and Your Life* (audio book). Sounds True.

Racey, Teri B., PA, MA. 2006. *Heart of Meditation, Guided Imagery for Deep Relaxation*. In the Mix.

————. 2008. *Master of the Storm, Life's Challenges Can Transform Your World*. In the Mix.

————. 2011. *New Body New Mind, A Guided Relaxation for Health and Happiness*. In the Mix.

Weil, Andrew, MD. 2001. *Meditation for Optimal Health: How to Use Mindfulness and Breathing to Heal* (audio book). Sounds True.

Websites

<u>www.12Step.com</u>

This website lists over fifty Twelve-Step programs. A Twelve-Step program is a community-based self-help group that uses twelve spiritually based action steps to help each individual become aware of and work to recover from dysfunctional/addictive thoughts and behaviors. These programs are donation based and focus on providing emotional support for individuals as they come to terms with various addictions such as alcohol, drugs, food, sex, gambling, depression, and other mental-health issues. The support is offered by those who are themselves in the recovery process. See the AA listing below as one representation of the many Twelve-Step programs available.

There are also many parallel programs for friends and family members to support them as they cope with their own thoughts and behaviors toward their addicted loved one. See the Al-Anon listing below as one representation of these support programs that are available.

<u>www.aa.com</u>

This is the official website for Alcoholics Anonymous, a Twelve-Step program for individuals struggling with alcohol use. Browse this site for information and meeting locations.

<u>www.al-anon.alateen.org</u>

Al-Anon is an organization for the friends and family of problem drinkers to help them cope more effectively. Browse this site for information and meeting locations.

Finding a Talk Therapist

Having an objective, skilled guide to help you explore and more effectively manage your challenge is immeasurably beneficial and also significantly reduces your recovery time.

Your choice of a talk therapist will and should be unique. It is dependent on what services are available in your community; your specific financial resources; and your belief system(s), medical needs, and social needs.

Tips for finding the right therapist for you

1. Compile a list of personal issues that are important to you in choosing a therapist. For example, you may feel more at ease talking to a therapist who is the same gender or who shares your religious or cultural beliefs.

2. Contact your medical-care center and/or medical-care practitioner(s) for their recommendations.

3. Ask trusted family and friends who have seen a talk therapist about their personal experiences. Word-of-mouth recommendations from those who have worked with a specific therapist are often most helpful.

4. Review your suggested list of therapists and see which ones will work with your insurance or current financial situation.

5. Make an appointment for an introductory visit during which you may distinguish if this particular therapist is a good fit for you.

6. Make a decision to create a dynamic, open partnership with your therapist so the self-discovery process can be most helpful and effective in addressing your goals and desires.

About the Author

Teri Battersby Racey, PA, MA, is a physician assistant with over three decades of clinical experience. Mindfulness meditation was the first nontraditional therapy Teri learned and then recommended to her patients. Teri found that those patients who practiced mindfulness meditation on a regular basis experienced significant reductions in their symptoms of anxiety, depression, insomnia, and physical pain. With regular meditation practice, their lives became more calm and peaceful. Even their relationships improved. These changes were so consistent and dramatic that Teri changed the entire focus of her clinical practice to teach mindfulness principles to individuals facing health or life challenges.

Supporting this change, Teri opened the Illumined Heart* in 2003. The Illumined Heart is dedicated to helping individuals achieve greater health of mind and body. Teri offers individual health consultations, classes, books, and CDs to support individuals in a desire for experiencing greater health and wellness.

Teri obtained a master's degree in Spirituality and Healing in Medicine from the University of Detroit Mercy, Detroit, Michigan. The focus of study explored how different cultural and belief systems may affect healing. A passionate advocate for preventive medicine, Teri taught health promotion coursework in the University of Detroit Mercy, Physician Assistant program.

Teri took the Professional Training Program in Mindfulness in Stress Reduction taught by Drs. Jon Kabat-Zinn and Saki Santorelli.

Teri's *New Mind New Body* guided relaxation CD provides a complement to this journal.

*The Illumined Heart logo invites individuals to walk their life path with an illumined heart and mind. A wise and compassionate heart and mind bring greater health and happiness to all who seek to represent themselves in this manner.

You may also enjoy Teri Racey's CDs and related items.

New Mind New Body (compact disc)

Master of the Storm (compact disc)

The Heart of Meditation (compact disc)

Dolphin Healing Journey (compact disc)

Purple Flame (compact disc)

"Walk Your Path with an Illumined Heart"
organic T-shirts and posters

"Love the Earth with All Your Heart"
organic T-shirts and posters